Lean and Green Cookbook for Beginners

The Perfect Cooking Plan to Start your Lean & Green Diet

Dwayne Copson

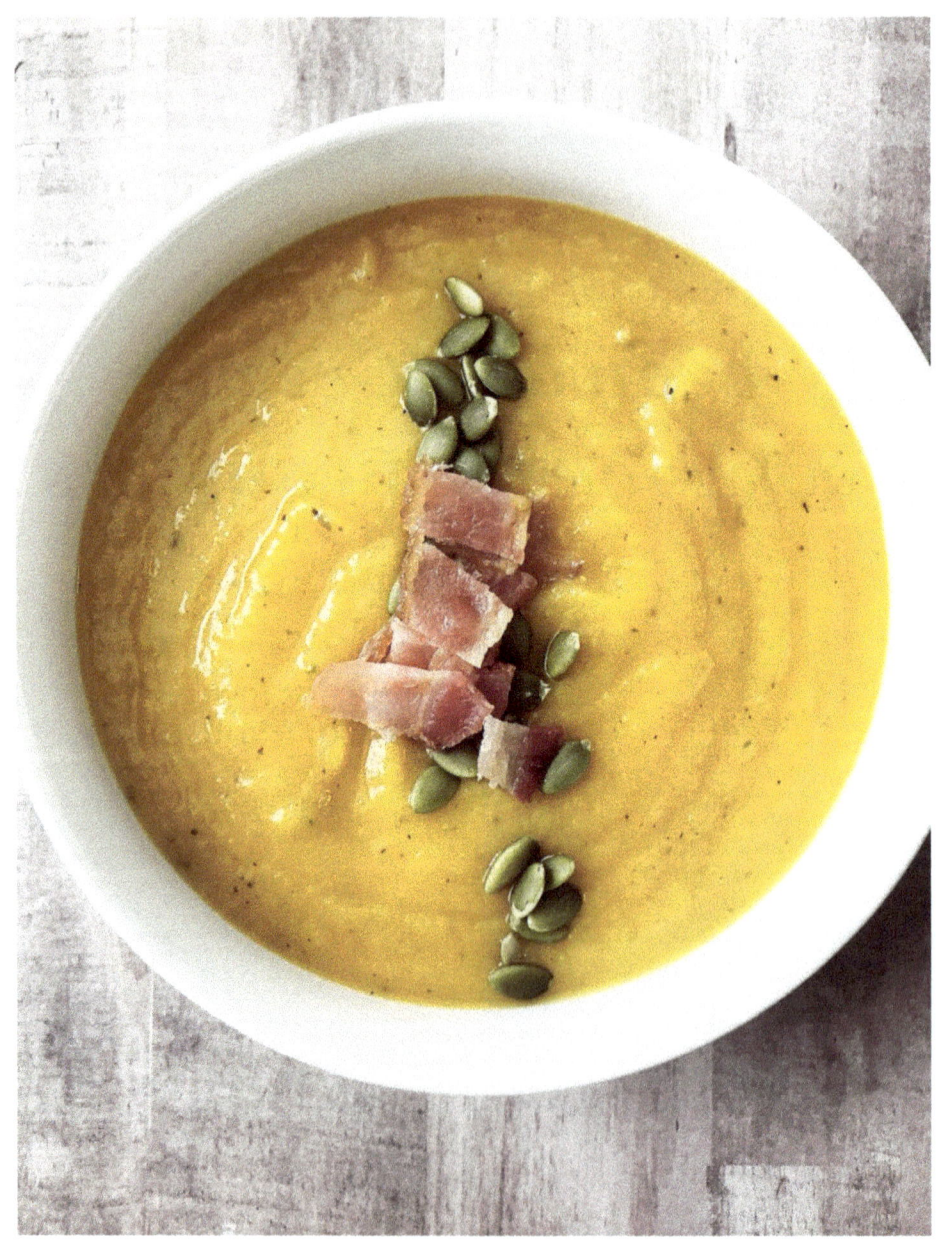

TABLE OF CONTENTS

Squash & Apple Soup

Servings: 6

Preparation time: 15 minutes

Cooking time: 8 hours

Ingredients:

- 5 cups of butternut squash, peeled and chopped
- 2 medium Granny Smith apples, peeled, cored and chopped
- 1 large carrot, peeled and chopped
- 1 small white onion, chopped
- 1 garlic clove, minced
- 4 cups of chicken broth
- 1 teaspoon of dried oregano, crushed
- 1 teaspoon of dried thyme, crushed
- Salt and ground black pepper, as required
- 1 cup of unsweetened coconut milk

Instructions:

1. In an oven-safe pan that will put in the Breville Smart Air Fryer Oven, add all Ingredients apart from coconut milk and stir to mix.
2. Cover the pan with a lid.
3. Arrange the pan over the wire rack.
4. Select "Slow Cooker" of Breville Smart Air Fryer Oven and assail "High".
5. Set the timer for 8 hours and press "Start/Stop" to start cooking.
1. 6 After 4½ hours of cocking, stir in the coconut milk and cheese.
2. 7 When the Cooking time is completed, remove the pan from the oven.
3. 8. Open the lid and stir in the coconut milk.
4. 9. With a stick blender, puree the soup until smooth.
5. 10. Serve immediately.

Chicken & Spinach Soup

Servings: 6

Preparation time: 15 minutes

Cooking time: 6 hours

Ingredients:

- 2 tablespoons of coconut oil, melted
- 4 cups of cooked chicken, chopped
- 8 cups of fresh spinach, chopped
- 1 large carrot, peeled and chopped
- 1 small onion, chopped finely
- ½ tablespoon of garlic, minced
- Salt and ground black pepper, as required
- 6 cups of low-sodium chicken broth

Instructions:

1. In an oven-safe pan that will put in the Breville Smart Air Fryer Oven, place all Ingredients and stir to mix.
2. Cover the pan with a lid.
3. Arrange the pan over the wire rack.

4. Select "Slow Cooker" of Breville Smart Air Fryer Oven and assail "Low".

5. Set the timer for six hours and press "Start/Stop" to start cooking.

6. When the Cooking time is completed, remove the pan from the oven.

7. Remove the lid and serve hot.

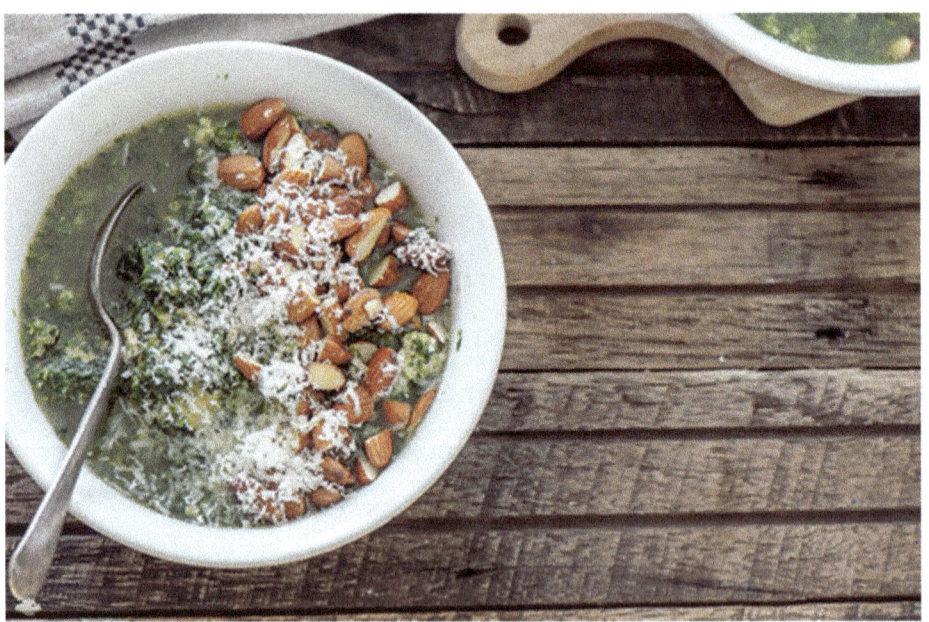

Chicken & Carrot Stew

Servings: 6

Preparation time: 15 minutes

Cooking time: 6 hours

Ingredients:

- 4 (5-ounce of) boneless chicken breast, cubed
- 3 cups of carrots, peeled and cubed
- 2 celery stalks, chopped
- 1 medium yellow onion, chopped
- 2 garlic cloves, minced
- Salt and ground black pepper, as required
- ½ teaspoon of dried thyme
- ½ teaspoon of dried rosemary
- 2 cups of chicken broth
- 2 tablespoons of olive oil

Instructions:

1. In an oven-safe pan that will put in the Breville Smart Air Fryer Oven, place all Ingredients apart from oil and stir to mix.

2. Cover the pan with a lid.

3. Arrange the pan over the wire rack.

4. Select "Slow Cooker" of Breville Smart Air Fryer Oven and assail "Low".

5. Set the timer for six hours and press "Start/Stop" to start cooking.

6. When the Cooking time is completed, remove the pan from the oven and serve hot.

7. Open the lid and stir in the oil.

8. Serve hot.

Turkey Meatballs & Spinach Soup

Servings: 6

Preparation time: 20 minutes

Cooking time: 6 hours 5 minutes

Ingredients:

For Meatballs:

- 2 pounds lean ground turkey
- 4 garlic cloves, minced
- ¼ cup of fresh cilantro, chopped
- 1 egg
- 2 teaspoons of dried rosemary, crushed
- Salt and ground black pepper, as required
- 2 tablespoons of olive oil

For Soup:

- 1 carrot, peeled and sliced large
- 1 large tomato, chopped
- 1 celery stalk, chopped
- 1 small onion, chopped

- Salt and ground black pepper, as required
- 7 cups of low-sodium chicken broth
- 6 cups of fresh spinach, chopped

Instructions:

1. For meatballs: in a large bowl, add all the Ingredients apart from oil and blend until well combined.
2. Make small sized balls from the mixture.
3. In a skillet, heat the oil over medium heat and cook the meatballs for about 4-5 minutes or until golden brown from all sides.
1. 4 With a slotted spoon, transfer the meatballs onto a plate.
2. 5 In an oven-safe pan that will put in the Breville Smart Air Fryer Oven, place the celery, onion, carrot and tomato.
6. Place the meatballs over the veggies.
7. Cover the pan with a lid.
8. Arrange the pan over the wire rack.
9. Select "Slow Cooker" of Breville Smart Air Fryer Oven and assail "Low".
10. Set the timer for six hours and press "Start/Stop" to start cooking.
11. When the Cooking time is completed, remove the pan from the oven and immediately, stir in the spinach.

12. Cover the pan with a lid for about 5 minutes before serving.

Cheesy Beef Soup

Servings: 8

Preparation time: 15 minutes

Cooking time: 5½ hours

Ingredients:

- 3 tablespoons of coconut oil
- 1 medium onion, chopped
- 2 celery stalks, chopped
- 2 large cloves garlic, minced
- 1-pound cooked beef, chopped
- 5 cups of low-sodium beef broth
- Salt and ground black pepper, as required 1 cup of full-fat coconut milk
- 1½ cups of low-fat Swiss cheese, shredded

Instructions:

1. In an oven-safe pan that will put in the Breville Smart Air Fryer Oven, melt the butter over medium heat and sauté the onion, celery and garlic and cook for about 5 minutes.

2. Stir in the beef, broth, salt and black pepper and take away from the heat.

3. Cover the pan with a lid.

4. Arrange the pan over the wire rack.

5. Select "Slow Cooker" of Breville Smart Air Fryer Oven and assail "High".

6. Set the timer for 5½ hours and press "Start/Stop" to start cooking.

7. After 4½ hours of cocking, stir in the coconut milk and cheese.

8. When the Cooking time is completed, remove the pan from the oven.

9. Open the lid and serve hot.

Beef Meatballs & Zucchini Soup

Servings: 8

Preparation time: 20 minutes

Cooking time: 6 hours 10 minutes

Ingredients:

For Meatballs:

- 2 pounds lean ground beef
- 4 garlic cloves, minced
- ¼ cup of fresh parsley leaves, chopped
- ½ cup of Parmesan cheese, grated
- 1 egg, beaten
- 1 teaspoon of dried oregano, crushed
- 1 teaspoon of dried rosemary, crushed
- Salt and ground black pepper, as required
- 2 tablespoons of coconut oil

For Soup:

- 1 celery stalk, chopped
- 1 small onion, chopped
- 1 small carrot, peeled and chopped
- 1 large plum tomato, chopped finely

- 3 large zucchinis, spiralized with a blade
- Salt and ground black pepper, as required
- 8 cups of low-sodium beef broth

Instructions:

1. For meatballs in a large bowl, add all Ingredients and blend until well combined.
2. Make small sized balls from the mixture.
3. In a large skillet, heat the oil over medium heat and cook the meatballs for about 4-5 minutes or until golden brown from all sides.
4. With a slotted spoon, transfer the meatballs onto a plate.
5. In an oven-safe pan that will put in the Breville Smart Air Fryer Oven, place the celery, onion, carrot and tomato.
6. Place the zucchini noodles over vegetables and sprinkle with salt and black pepper.
7. Place the broth over vegetables.
8. Carefully add meatballs in broth mixture.
9. Cover the pan with a lid.
10. Arrange the pan over the wire rack.
11. Select "Slow Cooker" of Breville Smart Air Fryer Oven and assail "Low".
12. Set the timer for six hours and press "Start/Stop" to start cooking.
13. When the Cooking time is completed, remove the pan from the oven and serve hot.

Ground Beef & Veggies Soup

Servings: 6

Preparation time: 15 minutes

Cooking time: 8¼ hours

Ingredients:

- 1 tablespoon of olive oil
- 1 yellow onion, chopped
- 2 garlic cloves, minced
- 1 teaspoon of dried oregano, crushed
- 1½ pounds ground beef
- 2 tomatoes, chopped
- 1 large zucchini, chopped
- 1 cup of fresh kale, tough ribs removed and chopped
- 5 cups of vegetable broth
- Salt and ground black pepper, as required

Instructions:

1. In an oven-safe pan that will put in the Breville Smart Air Fryer Oven, heat the oil over medium heat and sauté the onion for about 3-4 minutes.

2. Add the garlic and thyme and sauté for about 1 minute.

3. Add the meat and cook for about 4-5 minutes.

4. Add the tomatoes and cook for about 4-5 minutes.

5. Remove from the heat and stir in the remaining Ingredients.

6. Cover the pan with a lid.

7. Arrange the pan over the wire rack.

8. Select "Slow Cooker" of Breville Smart Air Fryer Oven and assail "Low".

9. Set the timer for 8 hours and press "Start/Stop" to start cooking.

10. When the Cooking time is completed, remove the pan from the oven.

11. Remove the lid and stir the mixture well.

12. Serve hot.

Beef & Cabbage Stew

Servings: 8

Preparation time: 15 minutes

Cooking time: 9 hours

Ingredients:

- 2 pounds beef stew meat, trimmed and cubed
- Salt and ground black pepper, as required
- 5 cups of green cabbage, chopped
- 1 large onion, chopped
- 6 garlic cloves, minced
- 4 medium fresh tomatoes, chopped
- 1 cup of beef broth
- 2 tablespoons of fresh parsley, chopped

Instructions:

1. In an oven-safe pan that will put in the Breville Smart Air Fryer Oven, place all Ingredients apart from parsley and stir to mix.
2. Cover the pan with a lid.
3. Arrange the pan over the wire rack.

4. Select "Slow Cooker" of Breville Smart Air Fryer Oven and assail "Low".

5. Set the timer for 9 hours and press "Start/Stop" to start cooking.

6. When the Cooking time is completed, remove the pan from the oven and serve hot.

7. Open the lid and serve hot with the garnishing of parsley.

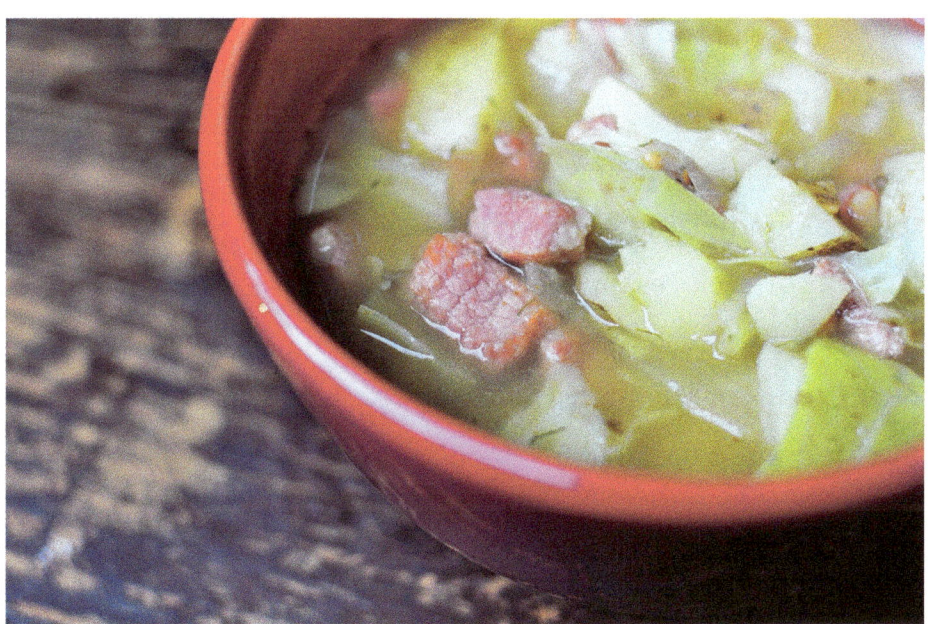

Beef & Mushroom Stew

Servings: 8

Preparation time: 15 minutes

Cooking time: 8 hours

Ingredients:

- 2 pounds beef stew meat, cubed
- 2 cups of fresh mushrooms, sliced
- 4 garlic cloves, minced
- 1 cup of fresh parsley leaves, chopped
- 2 cups of tomato paste
- 2 cups of beef broth
- Salt and ground black pepper, as required

Instructions:

1. In an oven-safe pan that will put in the Breville Smart Air Fryer Oven, place all Ingredients and stir to mix.
2. Cover the pan with a lid.
3. Arrange the pan over the wire rack.
4. Select "Slow Cooker" of Breville Smart Air Fryer Oven and assail "Low".

5. Set the timer for 8 hours and press "Start/Stop" to start cooking.
6. When the Cooking time is completed, remove the pan from the oven and serve hot.
7. Open the lid and serve hot.

Beef & Spinach Stew

Servings: 10

Preparation time: 15 minutes

Cooking time: 6 hours 10 minutes

Ingredients:

- ¼ cup of olive oil, divided
- 2½ pounds beef stew meat, cubed
- Salt and ground black pepper, as required
- 2 small onions, chopped
- 1 teaspoon of dried thyme, crushed
- 1 teaspoon of dried oregano, crushed
- 1 teaspoon of dried basil, crushed
- 1 cup of carrot, peeled and chopped
- 1 celery stalk, chopped
- 10 cups of fresh spinach, chopped
- 1 cup of fresh tomatoes, chopped finely
- 2 cups of chicken broth
- 3 tablespoons of fresh lemon juice

Instructions:

1. In an oven-safe pan that will put in the Breville Smart Air Fryer Oven, heat 2 tablespoons of the oil over medium heat and cook the meat cubes with salt and black pepper for about 4-5 minutes.
2. With a slotted spoon, transfer the meat cubes into a bowl.
3. In the pan, add the remaining oil and onions and cook for about 4-5 minutes.
4. Remove from the heat and stir in the cooked beef and remaining Ingredients apart from lemon juice.
5. Cover the pan with a lid.
6. Arrange the pan over the wire rack.
7. Select "Slow Cooker" of Breville Smart Air Fryer Oven and assail "Low".
8. Set the timer for six hours and press "Start/Stop" to start cooking.
9. When the Cooking time is completed, remove the pan from the oven and serve hot.
10. Open the lid and stir in the lemon juice.
11. Serve hot.

Pork & Cabbage Stew

Servings: 8

Preparation time: 15 minutes

Cooking time: 7½ hours

Ingredients:

- 2½ pounds boneless pork meat, cubed into 2-inch size
- 2½ cups of cabbage, chopped
- 2 cups of tomatoes, chopped finely
- 1 medium onion, chopped
- 2 garlic cloves, minced
- 2 tablespoons of olive oil
- 4 cups of chicken broth
- 1 tablespoon of fresh oregano, minced
- Salt and ground black pepper, as required
- 3 tablespoons of fresh lime juice

Instructions:

1. In an oven-safe pan that will put in the Breville Smart Air Fryer Oven, place all Ingredients and stir to mix.
2. Cover the pan with a lid.

3. Arrange the pan over the wire rack.
4. Select "Slow Cooker" of Breville Smart Air Fryer Oven and assail "Low".
5. Set the timer for 7½ hours and press "Start/Stop" to start cooking.
6. When the Cooking time is completed, remove the pan from the oven and serve hot.
7. Open the lid and transfer pork into a large bowl.
8. With 2 forks, shred the meat.
9. Return the shredded pork into the pan and blend well.
10. Serve hot with the drizzling of lemon juice.

Salmon & Veggie Stew

Servings: 4

Preparation time: 15 minutes

Cooking time: 6 hours

Ingredients:

- 1-pound salmon fillet, cubed
- 1 tablespoon of coconut oil
- 1 medium yellow onion, chopped
- 1 garlic clove, minced
- 1 zucchini, sliced
- 1 green bell pepper, seeded and cubed
- ½ cup of tomatoes, chopped
- ½ cup of fish broth
- ¼ teaspoon of dried oregano
- ¼ teaspoon of dried basil
- Salt and ground black pepper, as required

Instructions:

1. In an oven-safe pan that will put in the Breville Smart Air Fryer Oven, place all Ingredients and stir to mix.

2. Cover the pan with a lid.

3. Arrange the pan over the wire rack.

4. Select "Slow Cooker" of Breville Smart Air Fryer Oven and assail "Low".

5. Set the timer for 5-6 hours and press "Start/Stop" to start cooking.

6. When the Cooking time is completed, remove the pan from the oven and serve hot.

Seafood & Spinach Stew

Servings: 8

Preparation time: 20 minutes

Cooking time: 4 hours 50 minutes

Ingredients:

- 2 tablespoons of olive oil
- ½ pound tomatoes, chopped
- 1 large yellow onion, chopped finely
- 2 garlic cloves, minced
- 2 teaspoons of curry powder
- 6 sprigs fresh parsley
- Salt and ground black pepper, as required
- 1½ cups of chicken broth
- 1½ pounds salmon, cut into cubes
- 1½ pounds shrimp, peeled and deveined
- 1-pound fresh spinach, chopped

Instructions:

1. In an oven-safe pan that will put in the Breville Smart Air Fryer Oven, place all Ingredients apart from seafood and spinach and stir to mix.
2. Cover the pan with a lid.
3. Arrange the pan over the wire rack.
4. Select "Slow Cooker" of Breville Smart Air Fryer Oven and assail "Low".
5. Set the timer for 4 hours and press "Start/Stop" to start cooking.
6. When the Cooking time is completed, remove the pan from the oven.
7. Open the lid and stir in the seafood and spinach.
8. Cover the pan with a lid.
9. Arrange the pan over the wire rack.
10. Select "Slow Cooker" of Breville Smart Air Fryer Oven and assail "Low".
11. Set the timer for 50 minutes and press "Start/Stop" to start cooking.
12. When the Cooking time is completed, remove the pan from the oven and serve hot.

Herbed Seafood Stew

Servings: 8

Preparation time: 20 minutes

Cooking time: 4¾ hours

Ingredients:

- 1 small celery stalk, chopped
- 1 small carrot, peeled and chopped
- 1 yellow onion, chopped
- 3 garlic cloves, chopped
- 1 cup of fresh cilantro leaves, chopped
- 1 cup of tomatoes, chopped finely
- 4 cups of chicken broth
- 2 tablespoons of fresh lemon juice
- 2 tablespoons of olive oil
- 3 teaspoons of mixed dried herbs (rosemary, thyme, marjoram)
- Salt and ground black pepper, as required
- 1-pound cod fillets, cubed
- 1-pound shrimp, peeled and deveined
- 1-pound scallops
- ¾ cup of crabmeat

Instructions:

1. In an oven-safe pan that will put in the Breville Smart Air Fryer Oven, place all Ingredients apart from seafood and stir to mix.
2. Cover the pan with a lid.
3. Arrange the pan over the wire rack.
4. Select "Slow Cooker" of Breville Smart Air Fryer Oven and assail "Low".
5. Set the timer for 4 hours and press "Start/Stop" to start cooking.
6. When the Cooking time is completed, remove the pan from the oven.
7. Open the lid and stir in the seafood.
8. Cover the pan with a lid.
9. Arrange the pan over the wire rack.
10. Select "Slow Cooker" of Breville Smart Air Fryer Oven and assail "Low".
11. Set the timer for 45 minutes and press "Start/Stop" to start cooking.
12. When the Cooking time is completed, remove the pan from the oven and stir the mixture well.
13. Serve hot.

Spicy Chicken Legs

Servings: 6

Preparation time: 15 minutes

Cooking time: 25 minutes

Ingredients:

- 2½ pounds of chicken legs
- 2 tablespoons of olive oil
- 1 teaspoon of smoked paprika
- 1 teaspoon of garlic powder
- ½ teaspoon of ground cumin
- Salt and ground black pepper, as required
- 8 cups of fresh baby greens

Instructions:

1. In a large bowl, add all the Ingredients apart from baby greens and blend well.
2. Arrange the chicken legs onto the greased enamel roasting pan.
3. Select "Air Fry" of Breville Smart Air Fryer Oven and adjust the temperature to 400 degrees F.

4. Set the timer for 25 minutes and press "Start/Stop" to start preheating.

5. When the unit beeps to point out that it's preheated, insert the roasting pan in the oven.

6. When the Cooking time is completed, remove the roasting pan from the oven and transfer the chicken pieces onto a platter.

7. Serve hot alongside the baby greens.

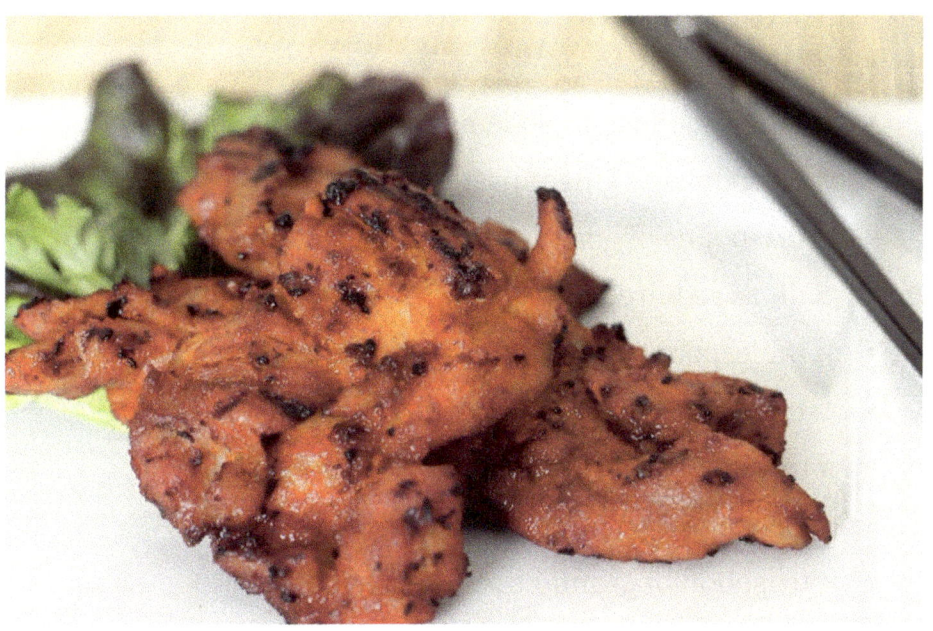

Marinated Chicken Legs

Servings: 4

Preparation time: 15 minutes

Cooking time: 20 minutes

Ingredients:

- 4 chicken legs
- 3 tablespoons of fresh lemon juice
- 3 teaspoons of ginger paste
- 3 teaspoons of garlic paste
- Salt, as required
- 4 tablespoons of low-fat plain yogurt
- 2 teaspoons of red chili powder
- 1 teaspoon of ground cumin
- 1 teaspoon of ground coriander
- 1 teaspoon of ground turmeric
- Ground black pepper, as required
- 6 cups of fresh baby kale

Instructions:

1. In a bowl, chicken legs, lemon juice, ginger paste, garlic paste, and salt and blend well.
2. Put aside for about 15 minutes.
3. Meanwhile, in another bowl, mix the yogurt, spices, and coloring.
4. Add the chicken legs into the bowl and generously coat with the spice mixture.
5. Cover the bowl of chicken and refrigerate for at least 10-12 hours.
6. Arrange the chicken legs into the greased air fry basket.
7. Select "Air Fry" of Breville Smart Air Fryer Oven and adjust the temperature to 445 degrees F.
8. Set the timer for 20 minutes and press "Start/Stop" to start preheating.
9. When the unit beeps to point out that it's preheated, insert the air fry basket in the oven.
10. When the Cooking time is completed, remove the air fry basket from the oven and serve hot alongside the kale.

Gingered Chicken Drumsticks

Servings: 3

Preparation time: 10 minutes

Cooking time: 25 minutes

Ingredients:

For Drumsticks:

- ¼ cup of full-fat coconut milk
- 2 teaspoons of fresh ginger, minced
- 2 teaspoons of galangal, minced
- 2 teaspoons of ground turmeric
- Salt, as required
- 3 (6-ounce of) chicken drumsticks

For Serving:

- 6 cups of fresh spinach

Instructions:

1. In a large bowl, add the coconut milk, galangal, ginger, and spices and blend well.

2. Add the chicken drumsticks and coat with the marinade generously.

3. Refrigerate to marinate for at least 6-8 hours.

4. Arrange the chicken drumsticks onto the greased enamel roasting pan.

5. Select "Air Fry" of Breville Smart Air Fryer Oven and adjust the temperature to 375 degrees F.

6. Set the timer for 25 minutes and press "Start/Stop" to start preheating.

7. When the unit beeps to point out that it's preheated, insert the roasting pan in the oven.

8. When the Cooking time is completed, remove the roasting pan from the oven and transfer the chicken drumsticks onto plates.

9. Serve hot alongside the spinach.

Chicken Casserole

Preparation time: 15 minutes

Cooking time: 40 minutes

Servings: 4

Ingredients:

- 1 lb. of cooked chicken; shredded
- ¼ cup of Greek yogurt
- 1 cup of cheddar cheese; shredded
- ½ cup of salsa
- 4 oz. of cream cheese; softened
- 4 cups of cauliflower florets
- 1/8 tsp. of black pepper
- ½ tsp. of kosher salt

Directions:

1. Add cauliflower florets into the microwave-safe dish and cook for 10 minutes or until soft.
2. Add cheese and microwave for 30 seconds more. Stir well.

3. Add chicken, yogurt, cheddar cheese, salsa, pepper, and salt and stir everything well.
4. Preheat the oven to 3750 F.
5. Bake in preheated oven for 20 minutes.
6. Serve hot and enjoy.

Nutrition:

- Calories: 429
- Fat: 23 g
- Carbs: 6 g
- Sugar: 7 g
- Protein: 44 g
- Cholesterol: 149 mg

Pressure Pot Chipotle Chicken & Cauliflower Rice Bowls

Preparation time: 10 minutes

Cooking time: 20 minutes

Servings: 4

Ingredients:

- 1/3 cup of salsa
- 1 quantity of 14.5 oz. of can fire-roasted diced tomatoes
- 1 canned chipotle pepper + 1 teaspoon sauce
- ½ teaspoon of dried oregano
- 1 teaspoon of cumin
- 1 ½ lb. of boneless, skinless chicken breast
- ¼ teaspoon of salt
- 1 cup of reduced-fat shredded Mexican cheese blend
- 4 cups of frozen diced cauliflower
- ½ medium-sized avocado, sliced

Directions:

1. Combine the primary Ingredients in a blender and blend until they become smooth.
2. Place the chicken in its pot and pour the sauce over it. Cover the lid and shut the pressure valve. Put it on high heat for 20 minutes. Allow the pressure release on its own before opening. Remove the chicken, and then add it back to the sauce.
3. Microwave the diced cauliflower according to the Directions on the package.
4. Before you serve, divide the diced cauliflower, cheese, avocado, and chicken equally among the 4 bowls.

Nutrition:

- Calories: 287
- Protein: 35 g
- Carbohydrate: 19 g
- Fat: 12 g

Tomato Cucumber Avocado Salad

Preparation time: 15 minutes

Cooking time: 0 minutes

Servings: 4

Ingredients:

- 12 oz. of cherry tomatoes, cut in half
- 5 small cucumbers; chopped
- 3 small avocados; chopped
- ½ tsp. of ground black pepper
- 2 tbsps. of olive oil
- 2 tbsps. of fresh lemon juice
- ¼ cup of fresh cilantro; chopped
- 1 tsp. of sea salt

Directions:

1. Add cherry tomatoes, cucumbers, avocados, and cilantro into the massive bowl and blend well.

2. Mix olive oil, lime juice, black pepper, and salt together and pour over the salad.

3. Toss well and serve immediately.

Nutrition:

- Calories: 442
- Fat: 31 g
- Carbs: 30.3 g
- Sugar: 4 g
- Protein: 2 g
- Cholesterol: 0 mg

Savory Cilantro Salmon

Preparation time: 10 minutes

Cooking time: 30 minutes

Servings: 4

Ingredients:

- 2 tablespoons of fresh lime or lemon
- 4 cups of fresh cilantro; divided
- 2 tablespoon of hot red pepper sauce
- ½ teaspoon of salt; divided
- 1 teaspoon of cumin
- 4, 7 oz. of salmon filets
- ½ cup of (4 oz.) water
- 2 cups of sliced red bell pepper
- 2 cups of sliced yellow bell pepper
- 2 cups of sliced green bell pepper
- Cooking spray
- ½ teaspoon of pepper

Directions:

1. Get a blender or food processor and mix half the cilantro, juice or lemon, cumin, hot red Poivrade, water, and salt; then puree until they become smooth. Transfer the marinade gotten into a large re-sealable bag.

2. Add salmon to marinade. Seal the bag, squeeze out air which may be trapped inside, add coat salmon. Refrigerate for about 1 hour, turning as often as possible.

3. Now, after marinating, preheat your oven to about 4000 F. Arrange the pepper slices in a single layer in a slightly greased, medium-sized square baking dish. Bake it for 20 minutes, then turn the pepper slices once.

4. Drain your salmon and do away with the marinade. Crust the upper part of the salmon with the remaining chopped, fresh cilantro. Place salmon on the top of the pepper slices and bake for about 12-14 minutes or until you notice that the fish flakes easily when it is tested with a fork. Enjoy.

Nutrition:

- Calories: 350
- Carbohydrate: 15 g
- Protein: 42 g
- Fat: 13 g

Chicken Zucchini Noodles

Preparation time: 20 minutes

Cooking time: 5 minutes

Servings: 2

Ingredients:

- 1 large zucchini, spiralized
- 1 chicken breast; skinless & boneless
- ½ tbsp. of jalapeno; minced
- 2 garlic cloves, minced
- ½ tsp. of ginger; minced
- ½ tbsp. fish sauce
- 2 tbsps. of coconut cream
- ½ tbsp. of honey
- ½ lime juice
- 1 tbsp. of peanut butter
- 1 carrot, chopped
- 2 tbsps. of cashews; chopped
- ¼ cup of fresh cilantro; chopped
- 1 tbsp. of olive oil
- Pepper

- Salt

Directions:

1. Heat vegetable oil in a pan over medium-high heat.
2. Season chicken breast with pepper and salt. Once the oil is hot then add chicken breast into the pan and cook for 3-4 minutes per side or until properly cooked.
3. Remove chicken breast from pan. Shred chicken breast with a fork and put aside.
4. In a small bowl, mix jalapeno, garlic, ginger, fish sauce, coconut milk, honey, and juice together. Set aside.
5. In a large bowl, combine together spiralized zucchini, carrots, cashews, cilantro, and shredded chicken.
6. Pour spread mixture over zucchini noodles and toss to mix.
7. Serve immediately and enjoy.

Nutrition:

- Calories 353
- Fat: 21 g
- Carbs: 20.5 g
- Sugar: 8 g
- Protein: 25 g
- Cholesterol: 54 mg

Lemon Garlic Oregano Chicken with Asparagus

Preparation time: 5 minutes

Cooking time: 40 minutes

Servings: 4

Ingredients:

- 1 small lemon, juiced (this should be about 2 tablespoons of lemon juice)
- 1 ¾ lb. of bone-in, skinless chicken thighs
- 2 tablespoon of fresh oregano, minced
- 2 cloves of garlic; minced
- 2 lbs. of asparagus; trimmed
- ¼ teaspoon each or less for black pepper and salt

Directions:

1. Preheat the oven to about 3500 F.
2. Put the chicken in a medium-sized bowl. Now, add the garlic, oregano, lemon juice, pepper, and salt and toss together to mix.

3. Roast the chicken in the air fryer oven until it reaches an indoor temperature of 1650 F in about 40 minutes. Once the chicken thighs are cooked, remove and keep aside to rest.
4. Now, steam the asparagus on a stovetop or in a microwave to the specified doneness.
5. Serve asparagus with the roasted chicken thighs.

Nutrition:

- Calories: 350
- Fat: 10 g
- Carbohydrate: 10 g
- Protein: 32 g

Healthy Broccoli Salad

Preparation time: 25 minutes

Cooking time: 0 minutes

Servings: 6

Ingredients:

- 3 cups of broccoli; chopped
- 1 tbsp. of apple cider vinegar
- ½ cup of Greek yogurt
- 2 tbsps. of sunflower seeds
- 3 bacon slices; cooked and chopped
- 1/3 cup of onion; sliced
- ¼ tsp. of stevia

Directions:

1. In a bowl, mix together broccoli, onion, and bacon.
2. In a small bowl, mix together yogurt, vinegar, stevia, and pour over the broccoli mixture. Stir to mix.
3. Sprinkle sunflower seeds on top of the salad.
4. Store salad in the refrigerator for 30 minutes.
5. Serve and enjoy.

Nutrition:

- Calories 90
- Fat: 9 g
- Carbs: 4 g
- Sugar: 5 g
- Protein: 2 g
- Cholesterol: 12 mg

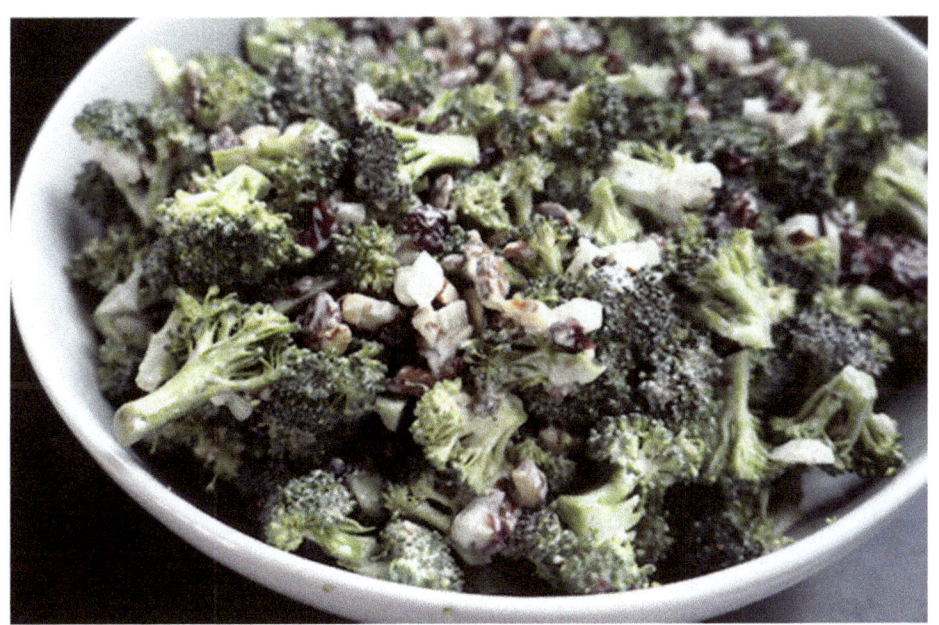

Parmesan Zucchini

Preparation time: 15 minutes

Cooking time: 15 minutes

Servings: 4

Ingredients:

- 4 zucchini; quartered lengthwise
- 2 tbsp. of fresh parsley; chopped
- 2 tbsps. of olive oil
- ¼ tsp. of garlic powder
- ½ tsp. of dried basil
- ½ tsp. of dried oregano
- ½ tsp. of dried thyme
- ½ cup of parmesan cheese; grated
- Pepper
- Salt

Directions:

1. Preheat the oven to 3500 F. Line baking sheet with parchment paper and put aside.

2. In a small bowl, mix together parmesan cheese, garlic powder, basil, oregano, thyme, pepper, and salt.
3. Arrange zucchini on the prepared baking sheet, drizzle with oil and sprinkle with parmesan cheese mixture.
4. Bake in preheated oven for 15 minutes then broil for 2 minutes or until lightly golden brown.
5. Garnish with parsley and serve immediately.

Nutrition:

- Calories: 244
- Fat: 14 g
- Carbs: 7 g
- Sugar: 5 g
- Protein: 15 g
- Cholesterol: 30 mg

Creamy Cauliflower Soup

Preparation time: 15 minutes

Cooking time: 15 minutes

Servings: 6

Ingredients:

- 5 cups of cauliflower rice
- 8 oz. of cheddar cheese; grated
- 2 cups of unsweetened almond milk
- 2 cups of vegetable stock
- 2 tbsps. of water
- 1 small onion; chopped
- 2 garlic cloves; minced
- 1 tbsp. of olive oil
- Pepper
- Salt

Directions:

1. Heat olive oil in a large stockpot over medium heat.
2. Add onion and garlic and cook for 1-2 minutes.

3. Add cauliflower rice and water. Cover and cook for 5-7 minutes.

4. Now add vegetable stock and almond milk and stir well. Bring to a boil.

5. Turn heat to low and simmer for five minutes.

6. Turn off the heat. Slowly add cheddar and stir until smooth.

7. Season soup with pepper and salt.

8. Stir well and serve hot.

Nutrition:

- Calories: 214
- Fat: 15 g
- Carbs: 3 g
- Sugar: 3 g
- Protein: 16 g
- Cholesterol: 40 mg

Sheet Pan Chicken Fajita Lettuce Wraps

Preparation time: 15 minutes

Cooking time: 30 minutes

Servings: 2

Ingredients:

- 1 lb. of chicken breast; thinly sliced into strips
- 2 teaspoons of olive oil
- 2 bell peppers; thinly sliced into strips
- 2 teaspoons of fajita seasoning
- 6 leaves from a romaine heart
- Juice of half a lime
- ¼ cup of plain of non-fat Greek yogurt

Directions:

1. Preheat your oven to about 4000 F.
2. Combine all of the Ingredients apart from lettuce in a large bag which will be resealed. Mix alright to coat vegetables and chicken with oil and seasoning evenly.

3. Spread the contents of the bag evenly on a foil-lined baking sheet. Bake it for about 25-30 minutes, or until the chicken is thoroughly cooked.

4. Serve on lettuce leaves and top with Greek yogurt if you wish.

Nutrition:

- Calories: 387
- Fat: 6 g
- Carbohydrate: 14 g
- Protein: 18 g

Taco Zucchini Boats

Preparation time: 20 minutes

Cooking time: 55 minutes

Servings: 4

Ingredients:

- 4 medium zucchinis; cut in half lengthwise
- ¼ cup of fresh cilantro; chopped
- ½ cup of cheddar cheese; shredded
- ¼ cup of water
- 4 oz. of tomato sauce
- 2 tbsps. of bell pepper; minced
- ½ small onion; minced
- ½ tsp. of oregano
- 1 tsp. of paprika
- 1 tsp. of chili powder
- 1 tsp. of cumin
- 1 tsp. of garlic powder
- 1 lb. of lean ground turkey
- ½ cup of salsa
- 1 tsp. of kosher salt

Directions:

1. Preheat the oven to 4000 F.
2. Add ¼ cup of salsa at the bottom of the baking dish.
3. Use a spoon to hollow the middle of the zucchini halves.
4. Chop the scooped-out flesh of zucchini and put aside ¾ of a cup chopped flesh.
5. Add zucchini halves in the boiling water and cook for 1 minute. Remove zucchini halves from water.
6. Add ground turkey in a large pan and cook until meat is no longer pink. Add spices and blend well.
7. Add the remaining zucchini halves, water, spaghetti sauce, bell pepper, and onion. Stir well and cover, then simmer over low heat for 20 minutes.
8. Stuff zucchini boats with taco meat and top each with one tablespoon of shredded cheddar.
9. Place zucchini boats in baking dish. Cover dish with foil and bake in preheated oven for 35 minutes.
10. Top with remaining salsa and chopped cilantro.
11. Serve and enjoy.

Nutrition:

- Calories: 297
- Fat: 17 g
- Carbs: 12 g
- Sugar: 3 g

- Protein: 30.2 g
- Cholesterol: 96 mg

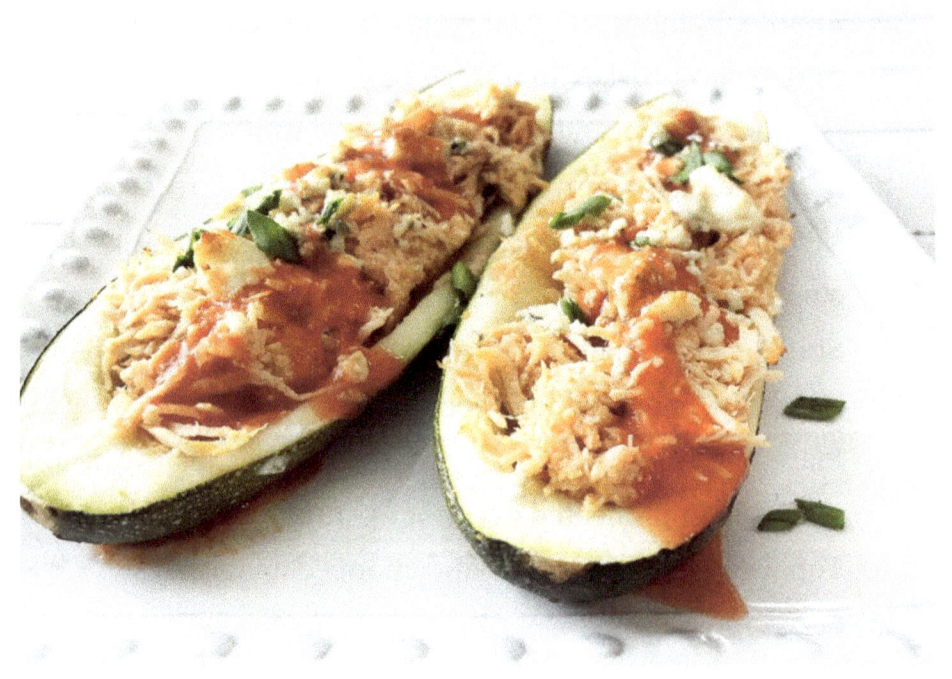

Cauliflower Rice

Preparation time: 5 minutes

Cooking time: 20 minutes

Servings: 1

Ingredients:

Round 1:

- 1/2 tsp. of turmeric
- 1/2 cup of diced carrot
- 1/8 cup of diced onion
- 1/2 tbsp. of low-sodium soy sauce
- 1/8 block of extra firm tofu

Round 2:

- 1/2 cup of frozen peas
- 1/4 minced garlic cloves
- 1/2 cup of chopped broccoli
- 1/2 tbsp. of minced ginger
- 1/4 tbsp. of rice vinegar
- 1/4 tsp. of toasted sesame oil
- 1/2 tbsp. of reduced-sodium soy sauce
- 1/2 cup of diced cauliflower

Directions:

1. Crush tofu in a large bowl and toss with all the Round one ingredient.

2. Lock the air fryer lid—preheat the instant crisp airfryer to 3700 F. Also, set the temperature to 370°F, set time to 10 minutes, and cook for 10 minutes, making sure to shake once.

3. In another bowl, toss Ingredients from Round 2 together.

4. Add Round 2 mixture to instant crisp airfryer and cook for another 5 to 10 minutes.

5. Enjoy!

Nutrition:

- Calories: 67
- Fat: 8 g
- Protein: 3 g
- Sugar: 0 g

Great Lunch Omelet

Preparation time: 5 minutes

Cooking time: 10 minutes

Servings: 2

Ingredients:

- 4 medium mushrooms; sliced, 2 oz.
- 1 green onion; sliced
- 2 eggs; beaten
- 1 oz. of Jarlsberg or Swiss cheese; shredded
- 1 oz. of ham; diced

Directions:

1. In a skillet, cook the mushrooms and scallion until soft.
2. Add the eggs and blend well.
3. Sprinkle with salt and top with the mushroom mixture, cheese, and the ham.
4. When the egg is settled, fold the plain side of the omelet on the filled side.
5. Turn off the heat and let it stand until the cheese has melted.

6. Serve!

Nutrition:

- Calories: 288
- Carbs: 22 g
- Fat: 12 g
- Protein: 27 g
- Fiber: 6 g

Stuffed Mushrooms

Preparation time: 7 minutes

Cooking time: 8 minutes

Servings: 1

Ingredients:

- 1/2 rashers bacon; diced
- 1/2 onion; diced
- 1/2 bell pepper; diced
- 1/2 small carrot; diced
- 2 medium size mushrooms (separate the caps and stalks)
- 1/4 cup of shredded cheddar plus extra for two top
- 1/4 cup of sour cream

Directions:

1. Chop the mushrooms stalks finely and fry them up with the bacon, onion, pepper, and carrot at 350°F for 8 minutes.

2. Also, check when the veggies are soft, and stir in the soured cream and the cheese. Keep up the heat until the cheese has melted, and everything is mixed nicely.
3. Now grab the mushroom caps and heap a plop of filling on all.
4. Place in the fryer basket and top with a little extra cheese.

Nutrition:

- Calories: 285
- Fat: 20.5 g
- Protein: 8.6 g

Jalapeno Cheese Balls

Preparation time: 10 minutes

Cooking time: 8 minutes

Servings: 1

Ingredients:

- 1-ounce of cream cheese
- 1/6 cup of shredded mozzarella cheese
- 1/6 cup of shredded Cheddar cheese
- 1/2 jalapeños; finely chopped
- 1/2 cup of breadcrumbs
- 2 eggs
- 1/2 cup of all-purpose flour
- Salt
- Pepper
- Cooking oil

Directions:

1. Mix the cream cheese, mozzarella, Cheddar cheese, and jalapeños in a medium bowl. Mix very well.

2. Form the cheese mixture into balls about an inch thick. You can also use a little ice cream scoop. It works well.

3. Arrange the cheese balls on a sheet pan and place in the freezer for 15 minutes. It can help the cheese balls maintain their shape while frying.

4. Spray the instant Crisp Air Fryer basket with olive oil.

5. Place the breadcrumbs in a small bowl. Beat the eggs in another small bowl. In a third small bowl, mix the flour with salt and pepper to taste, and blend well.

6. Remove the cheese balls from the freezer. Plunge the cheese balls in the flour, then the eggs, then the breadcrumbs.

7. Place the cheese balls in the Instant Crisp Air Fryer. Spray with olive oil. Lock the air fryer lid. Cook for 8 minutes.

8. Open the instant Crisp Air Fryer and flip the cheese balls. I would like to recommend flipping them rather than shaking, so the balls maintain their form. Cook for more 4 minutes.

9. Cool before serving.

Nutrition:

- Calories: 96
- Fat: 6 g
- Protein: 4 g
- Sugar: 0 g

Zucchini Omelet

Preparation time: 10 minutes

Cooking time: 10 minutes

Servings: 1

Ingredients:

- 1/2 teaspoon of butter
- 1/2 zucchini; julienned
- 1 egg
- 1/8 teaspoon of fresh basil; chopped
- 1/8 teaspoon of red pepper flakes, crushed
- Salt and newly ground black pepper, to taste

Directions:

1. Preheat the instant Crisp Air Fryer to 3550 F.
2. Melt butter on a medium heat using a skillet.
3. Add zucchini and cook for about 3-4 minutes.
4. In a bowl, add the eggs, basil, red pepper flakes, salt, black pepper, and beat well.
5. Add cooked zucchini and gently stir to mix.

6. Transfer the mixture into the instant Crisp Air Fryer pan. Lock the air fryer lid.

7. Cook for about 10 minutes. Also, you might prefer to wait until it is thoroughly done.

Nutrition:

- Calories: 285
- Fat: 20.5 g
- Protein: 8.6 g

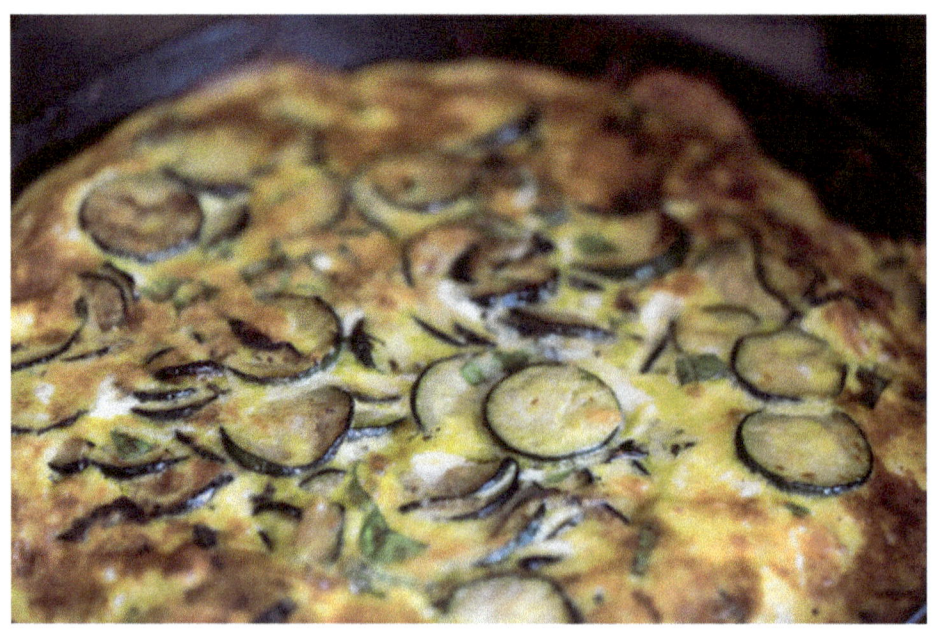

Courgette Risotto

Preparation time: 10 minutes

Cooking time: 5 minutes

Servings: 8

Ingredients:

- 2 tablespoons of olive oil
- 4 cloves garlic; finely chopped
- 1.5 pounds of Arborio rice
- 6 tomatoes; chopped
- 2 teaspoons of chopped rosemary
- 6 courgettes; finely diced
- 1 ¼ cups of peas; fresh or frozen
- 12 cups of hot vegetable stock
- Salt to taste
- Freshly ground pepper

Directions:

1. Place a large, heavy-bottomed pan over medium heat. Add oil. When the oil is heated, add onion and sauté until translucent.

2. Stir in the tomatoes and cook until soft.

3. Stir in the rice and rosemary. Mix well.

4. Add half the stock and cook until dry. Stir frequently.

5. Add remaining stock and cook for 3-4 minutes.

6. Add courgette and peas and cook until rice becomes soft. Add salt and pepper to taste.

7. Stir in the basil. Let it sit for 5 minutes.

Nutrition:

- Calories: 406
- Fats: 5 g
- Carbohydrates: 82 g
- Proteins: 14 g

Cheesy Cauliflower Fritters

Preparation time: 10 minutes

Cooking time: 7 minutes

Servings: 1

Ingredients:

- 1/2 cup of chopped parsley
- 1 cup of Italian breadcrumbs
- 1/3 cup of shredded mozzarella cheese
- 1/3 cup of shredded sharp cheddar cheese
- 1 egg
- 2 minced garlic cloves
- 3 chopped scallions
- 1 head of cauliflower

Directions:

1. Cut the cauliflower up into florets. Wash well and pat dry. Place into a food processor and pulse for 20-30 seconds or till it's like rice.

2. Place the cauliflower rice in a bowl and blend with pepper, salt, egg, cheeses, breadcrumbs, garlic, and scallions.

3. Make 15 patties of the mixture with hands, then add more breadcrumbs if needed.

4. Spritz patties with vegetable oil, and put the fitters into your Instant Crisp Air Fryer. Pile it in a single layer. Lock the air fryer lid. Set temperature to 390°F, and set time to 7 minutes, flipping after 7 minutes.

Nutrition:

- Calories: 209
- Fat: 17 g
- Protein: 6 g
- Sugar: 0.5 g

Bell-Pepper Corn Wrapped in Tortilla

Preparation time: 5 minutes

Cooking time: 15 minutes

Servings: 1

Ingredients:

- 1/4 small red bell pepper; chopped
- 1/4 small yellow onion; diced
- 1/4 tablespoon of water
- 1/2 cob of grilled corn kernels
- 1 large tortilla
- One-piece commercial vegan nuggets, chopped
- Mixed greens for garnish

Directions:

1. Preheat the Crisp Air Fryer to 400°F.
2. In a skillet heated over medium heat, sauté the vegan nuggets, onions, bell peppers, and corn kernels. Set aside.
3. Place filling inside the corn tortillas.

4. Lock the air fryer lid. Fold the tortillas and place inside the moment Crisp Air Fryer. Cook for 15 minutes or until the tortilla wraps are crispy.
5. Serve with mixed greens on top.

Nutrition:

- Calories: 548
- Fat: 20.7 g
- Protein: 46 g

Zucchini Parmesan Chips

Preparation time: 10 minutes

Cooking time: 8 minutes

Servings: 1

Ingredients:

- 1/2 tsp. of paprika
- 1/2 cup of grated parmesan cheese
- 1/2 cup of Italian breadcrumbs
- 1 lightly beaten egg
- 2 thinly sliced zucchinis

Directions:

1. Use a really sharp knife or mandolin slicer to slice the zucchini as thinly as you can. Pat off extra moisture.
2. Beat the egg with a pinch of pepper, salt, and a bit of water.
3. Combine paprika, cheese, and breadcrumbs in a bowl.
4. Dip slices of zucchini into the egg mixture and then into breadcrumb mixture. Press gently to coat.

5. Mist encrusted zucchini slices with vegetable oil cooking spray. Put them into your Instant Crisp Air Fryer in a single layer. Latch the air fryer lid. Set temperature to 350°F and set time to 8 minutes.
6. Sprinkle with salt and serve with salsa.

Nutrition:

- Calories: 211
- Fat: 16 g
- Protein: 8 g
- Sugar: 0 g

Prosciutto Spinach Salad

Preparation time: 5 minutes

Cooking time: 5 minutes

Servings: 2

Ingredients:

- 2 cups of baby spinach
- 1/3 lb. of prosciutto
- 1 cantaloupe
- 1 avocado
- ¼ cup of diced red onion
- Handful of raw, unsalted walnuts

Directions:

1. Put a cup of spinach on each plate.
2. Top with the diced prosciutto, cubes of melon, slices of avocado, a couple of purple onion, and a couple of walnuts.
3. Add some freshly ground pepper, if you wish.
4. Serve!

Nutrition:

- Calories: 348
- Carbs: 11 g
- Fat: 9 g
- Protein: 26 g
- Fiber: 22 g

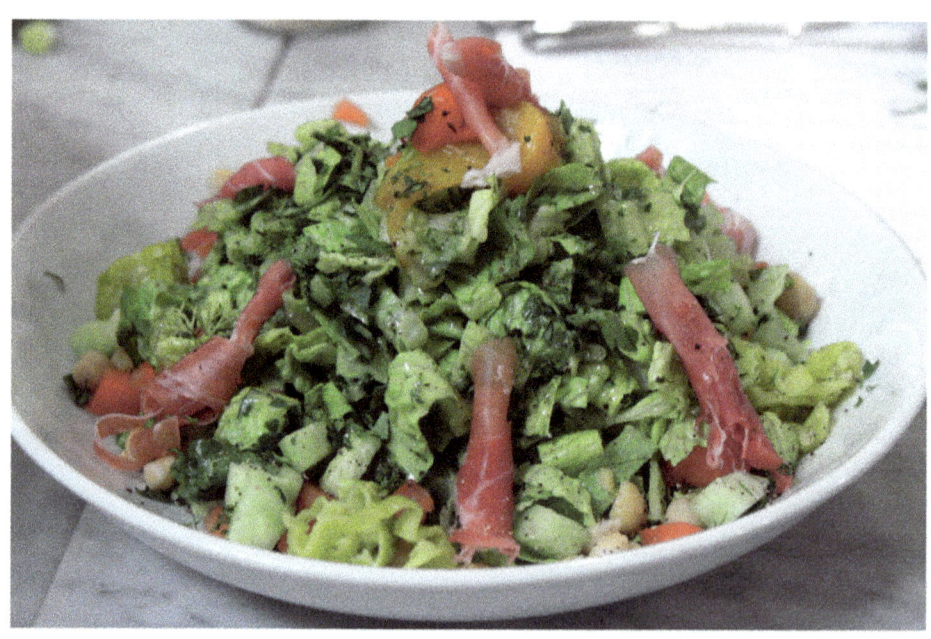

Crispy Roasted Broccoli

Preparation time: 10 minutes

Cooking time: 8 minutes

Servings: 1

Ingredients:

- 1/4 tsp. of Masala
- 1/2 tsp. of red chili powder
- 1/2 tsp. of salt
- 1/4 tsp. of turmeric powder
- 1 tbsp. of chickpea flour
- 1 tbsp. of yogurt
- 1/2-pound of broccoli

Directions:

1. Cut broccoli up into florets. Immerse in a bowl of water with two teaspoons of salt for at least half an hour to get rid of impurities.
2. Take out broccoli florets from water and allow to drain. Wipe down thoroughly.
3. Mix all other Ingredients to make a marinade.

4. Toss broccoli florets into the marinade. Cover and chill for 15-30 minutes.

5. Preheat the instant Crisp Air Fryer to 3900 F. Place marinated broccoli florets into the fryer, lock the air fryer lid, set the temperature to 350°F, and set time to 10 minutes. Florets are going to be crispy when done.

Nutrition:

- Calories: 96
- Fat: 1.3 g
- Protein: 7 g
- Sugar: 4.5 g

Grilled Ham & Cheese

Preparation time: 15 minutes

Cooking time: 30 minutes

Servings: 2

Ingredients:

- 3 low-carb buns
- 4 slices of medium-cut deli ham
- 1 tbsp. of salted butter
- 1 oz. of flour
- 3 slices of cheddar cheese
- 3 slices of muenster cheese

Directions:

Bread:

1. Preheat your fryer to 350°F/175°C.
2. Mix the flour, salt, and baking powder in a bowl. Set aside.
3. Add in the butter and coconut oil to a skillet.
4. Melt for 20 seconds and pour into another bowl.
5. In this bowl, mix in the dough.

6. Scramble 2 eggs and add to the dough.
7. Add ½ tablespoon of coconut flour to thicken, and place evenly in a cupcake tray. Fill about ¾ inch.
8. Bake for 20 minutes or until browned.
9. Allow to chill for 15 minutes and cut each in half for the buns.

Sandwich:

10. Fry the deli meat in a skillet on a high heat.
11. Put the ham and cheese between the buns.
12. Heat the butter on medium-high.
13. When brown, turn heat to low and add the dough to the pan.
14. Press down with a weight until you smell burning, then flip to crisp each side.
15. Enjoy!

Nutrition:

- Calories: 188
- Carbs: 12 g
- Fat: 16 g
- Protein: 14 g
- Fiber: 18 g

Coconut Battered Cauliflower Bites

Preparation time: 5 minutes

Cooking time: 20 minutes

Servings: 1

Ingredients:

- Salt and pepper to taste
- 1 flax egg or 1 tablespoon flaxseed meal + 3 tablespoons of water
- 1 small cauliflower; cut into florets
- 1 teaspoon of mixed spice
- 1/2 teaspoon of mustard powder
- 2 tablespoons of maple syrup
- 1 clove of garlic; minced
- 2 tablespoons of soy sauce
- 1/3 cup of oats flour
- 1/3 cup of plain flour
- 1/3 cup of desiccated coconut

Directions:

1. In a bowl, mix oats, flour, and desiccated coconut. Season with salt and pepper to taste, then set aside.
2. Place the flax egg in another bowl and add a pinch of salt to taste. Set aside.
3. Season the cauliflower with mixed spice and mustard powder.
4. Dredge the florets in the flax egg first, then in the flour mixture.
5. Place it inside the instant Crisp Air Fryer, lock the air fryer lid, and cook at 400°F for 15 minutes.
6. Meanwhile, place the maple syrup, garlic, and soy in a saucepan and heat over medium flame. Wait for it to boil and adjust the heat to low until the sauce thickens.
7. After 15 minutes, remove the florets inside the instant Crisp Air Fryer and place them in the saucepan.
8. Toss to coat the florets, then place them inside the instant Crisp Air Fryer and cook for an additional 5 minutes.

Nutrition:

- Calories: 154
- Fat: 2.3 g
- Protein: 4.69 g

Mashed Garlic Turnips

Preparation time: 5 minutes

Cooking time: 10 minutes

Servings: 2

Ingredients:

- 3 cups of diced turnip
- 2 cloves of garlic; minced
- ¼ cup of heavy cream
- 3 tbsps. of melted butter
- Salt and pepper to season

Directions:

1. Boil the turnips until it is soft.
2. Drain and mash the turnips.
3. Add the cream, butter, salt, pepper and garlic. Mix very well.
4. Serve!

Nutrition:

- Calories: 488
- Carbs: 32 g
- Fat: 19 g
- Protein: 34 g
- Fiber: 20 g

Air Fryer Asparagus

Preparation time: 5 minutes

Cooking time: 8 minutes

Servings: 1

Ingredients:

- Nutritional yeast
- Olive oil non-stick spray
- 1 bunch of asparagus

Directions:

1. Wash the asparagus. Don't forget to trim off the thick, woody ends.
2. Spray with olive oil spray and sprinkle with yeast.
3. In your Instant Crisp Air Fryer, lay the asparagus in a singular layer. Set the temperature to 360°F. Set the time to 8 minutes.

Nutrition:

- Calories: 17

- Fat: 4 g
- Protein: 9 g

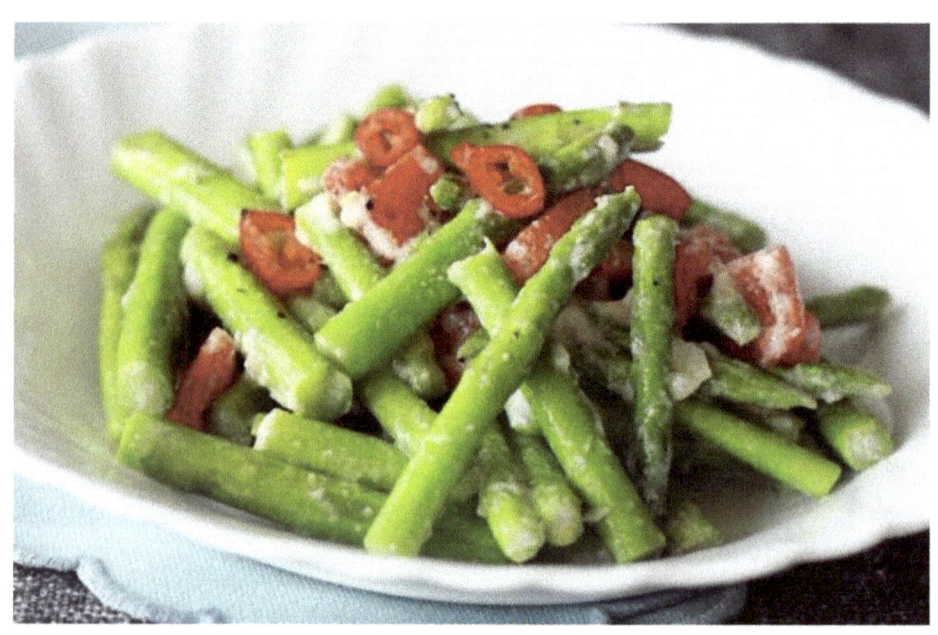

Avocado Fries

Preparation time: 10 minutes

Cooking time: 7 minutes

Servings: 1

Ingredients:

- 1 avocado
- 1/8 tsp. of salt
- 1/4 cup of panko breadcrumbs
- Bean liquid (aquafaba) from a 15-ounce can of white or garbanzo beans

Directions:

1. Peel, pit, and slice avocado.
2. Toss salt and breadcrumbs together in a bowl. Place the aquafaba into another bowl.
3. Dredge slices of avocado first in the aquafaba then in the panko, ensuring you are evenly coating.
4. Place coated avocado slices into one layer in the Instant Crisp Air Fryer. Set temperature to 390°F and set time to 5 minutes.

5. Serve with your favorite Keto dipping sauce!

Nutrition:

- Calories: 102
- Fat: 22 g
- Protein: 9 g
- Sugar: 1 g

Diced Cauliflower & Curry Chicken

Preparation time: 15 minutes

Cooking time: 30 minutes

Servings: 6

Ingredients:

- 2 lbs. of chicken (4 breasts)
- 1 packet of curry paste
- 3 tbsps. of ghee (can substitute with butter)
- ½ cup of heavy cream
- 1 head of cauliflower (around 1 kg)

Directions:

1. In a large skillet, melt the ghee.
2. Add the curry paste and blend.
3. Once mixed, add a cup of water and simmer for 5 minutes.
4. Add the chicken, cover the skillet and simmer for 18 minutes.

5. Cut a cauliflower head into florets and blend in a food processor to form the diced cauliflower.
6. When the chicken is cooked, uncover, add the cream and cook for more 7 minutes.
7. Serve!

Nutrition:

- Calories: 267
- Carbs: 42 g
- Fat: 31 g
- Protein: 34 g
- Fiber: 32 g

Jalapeno Coins

Preparation time: 10 minutes

Cooking time: 5 minutes

Servings: 1

Ingredients:

- 1 egg
- 2/3 tbsp. of coconut flour
- 1 sliced and seeded jalapeno
- Pinch of garlic powder
- Pinch of onion powder
- Bit of Cajun seasoning (optional)
- Pinch of pepper and salt

Directions:

1. Ensure your Instant Crisp Air Fryer is preheated to 4000 F.
2. Mix all dry Ingredients.
3. Pat jalapeno slices dry. Dip them into the egg wash, and then into the dry mixture. Toss to coat thoroughly.

4. Add coated jalapeno slices to Instant Crisp Air Fryer in a singular layer. Spray with vegetable oil.

5. Lock the air fryer lid. Set temperature to 350°F and set time to 5 minutes. Cook till just crispy.

Nutrition:

- Calories: 128
- Fat: 8 g
- Protein: 7 g
- Sugar: 0 g

Lasagna Spaghetti Squash

Preparation time: 30 minutes

Cooking time: 90 minutes

Servings: 6

Ingredients:

- 25 slices of mozzarella cheese
- 1 large jar (40 oz.) of Rao's Marinara sauce
- 30 oz. of whole-milk ricotta cheese
- 2 large spaghetti squash; cooked (44 oz.)
- 4 lbs. of ground beef

Directions:

1. Preheat your fryer to 375°F/190°C.
2. Slice the spaghetti squash and place it face down inside a fryer proof dish. Fill with water until covered.
3. Heat for 45 minutes or until the skin is soft.
4. Roast the meat until it browns.
5. In a large skillet, heat the browned meat and marinara sauce. Put aside when warm.

6. Scrape the flesh off the cooked squash to resemble strands of spaghetti.
7. Layer the lasagna in a large greased pan in alternating layers of spaghetti squash, meat sauce, mozzarella, and ricotta. Repeat until all are layered.
8. Bake for 30 minutes and serve!

Nutrition:

- Calories: 508
- Carbs: 32 g
- Fat: 8 g
- Protein: 22 g
- Fiber: 21 g

Monkey Salad

Preparation time: 4 minutes

Cooking time: 7 minutes

Servings: 1

Ingredients:

- 2 tbsps. of butter
- 1 cup of unsweetened coconut flakes
- 1 cup of raw, unsalted cashews
- 1 cup of 90% dark chocolate shavings

Directions:

1. In a skillet, melt the butter on a medium heat.
2. Add the coconut flakes and sauté until it becomes lightly browned or for 4 minutes.
3. Add the cashews and sauté for 3 minutes. Remove from the heat and sprinkle with bittersweet chocolate shavings.
4. Serve!

Nutrition:

- Calories: 321
- Carbs: 5 g
- Fat: 12 g
- Protein: 6 g
- Fiber: 5 g

Mu Shu Lunch Pork

Preparation time: 5 minutes

Cooking time: 10 minutes

Servings: 2

Ingredients:

- 4 cups of coleslaw mix, with carrots
- 1 small onion; sliced thin
- 1 lb. of cooked roast pork; cut into ½" cubes
- 2 tbsps. of hoisin sauce
- 2 tbsps. of soy sauce

Directions:

1. In a large skillet, heat the oil on high heat.
2. Stir-fry the cabbage and onion for 4 minutes or until they are soft.
3. Add the pork, hoisin, and soy sauce.
4. Cook until browned.
5. Enjoy!

Nutrition:

- Calories: 388
- Carbs: 16 g
- Fat: 21 g
- Protein: 25 g
- Fiber: 16 g

Fiery Jalapeno Poppers

Preparation time: 10 minutes

Cooking time: 40 minutes

Servings: 4

Ingredients:

- 5 oz. of cream cheese
- ¼ cup of mozzarella cheese
- 8 medium jalapeno peppers
- ½ tsp. of Mrs. Dash Table Blend
- 8 slices of bacon

Directions:

1. Preheat your fryer to 400°F/200°C.
2. Cut the jalapenos in half.
3. Use a spoon to scrape out the insides of the peppers.
4. In a bowl, mix together the cream cheese, mozzarella cheese and spices of your choice.
5. Pack the cheese mixture into the jalapenos and place the peppers on top.
6. Wrap each pepper in 1 slice of bacon, from bottom to top.

7. Bake for 30 minutes. Broil for a further 3 minutes.
8. Serve!

Nutrition:

- Calories: 238
- Carbs: 4 g
- Fat: 10 g
- Protein: 24 g
- Fiber: 14 g

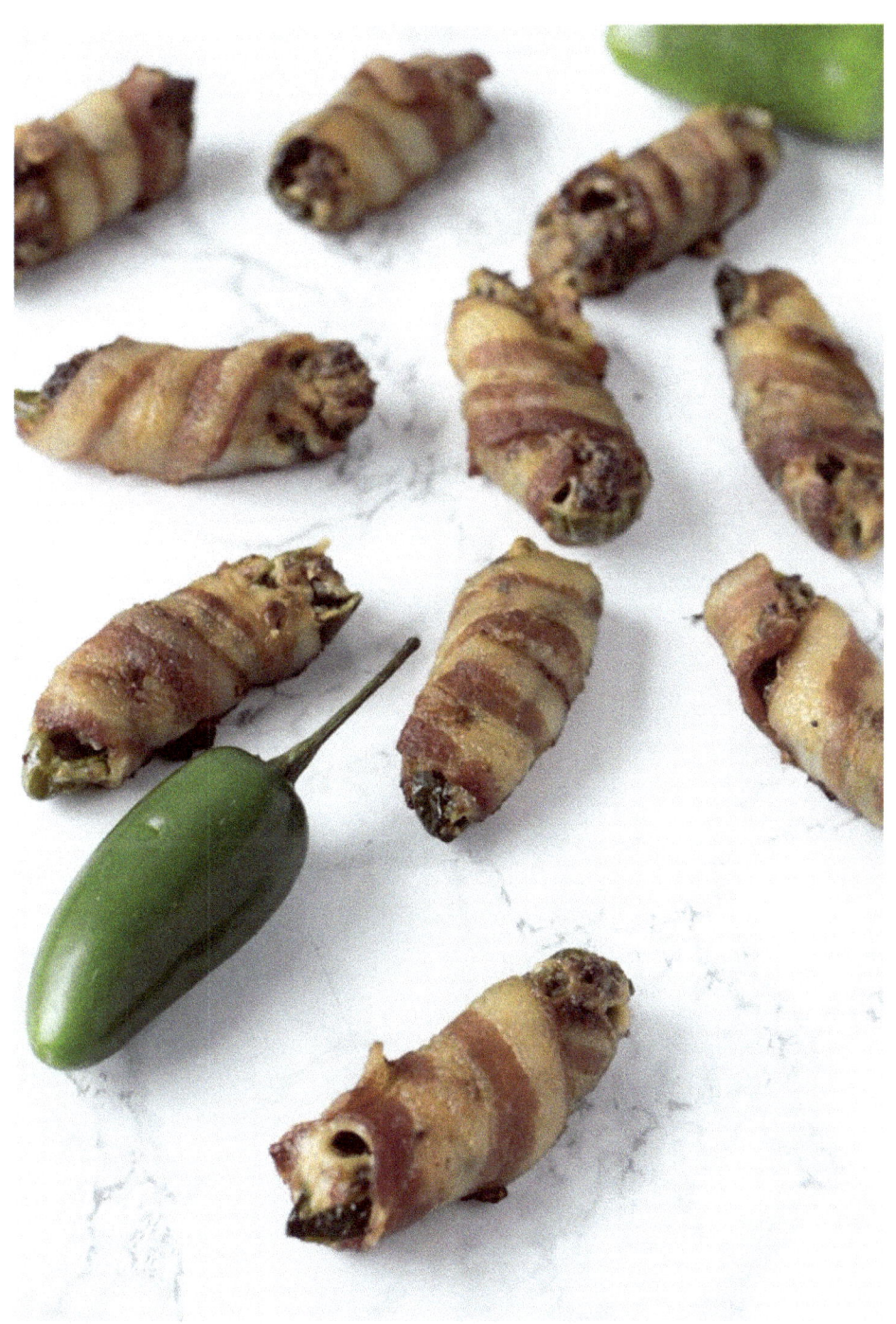

Lightning Source UK Ltd.
Milton Keynes UK
UKHW020636140621
385477UK00005B/95